FIRST MOON

WELCOME TO WOMANHOOD

ANKE MAI

Praise for the
First Edition (2000)

"My daughter loves First Moon and keeps it by her bed. She hasn't started bleeding yet, but is looking forward to it very much."

"An oasis in the desert of celebrating menarche."

"I read this book with delight. I think it is wonderful, and such an important topic, covered so creatively, thoughtfully, and comprehensively."

"I shall keep your book as a treasure."

"Your book is very nicely done, and totally targets the age group of the prepubescent girl. I can't wait to share it."

"I have been delighted with First Moon and refer back to it often for ideas in my work as a Menstrual Health Educator. Thank you for your inspiration."

"Your contribution to change has been immense."

"This book deserves to be required reading for every girl aged ten and over."

Praise for the Current Edition

Anke Mai's First Moon book has had a huge influence on women for two decades, helping and empowering us to stand together with our daughters in support and kindness, and deepening our understanding of what it means to be a woman. This wonderful book is a rich mixture of really solid information every girl needs to know and a deeper wisdom, connection and empowerment every girl needs to develop, to become a wise woman. Its significance is far-reaching and I thank Anke Mai from the bottom of my heart for this great gift she has given us all.

Glennie Kindred, author of many books on celebrating ourselves and the Earth, www.glenniekindred.co.uk

As women we are hungry for information to help our daughters and granddaughters to have access to information that wasn't available to us as we grew up.

In Goddess Temple Gifts, we sell many First Moon books to women who are hungry for ways to speak to their daughters and granddaughters about this very special, once in a lifetime experience. First Moon is a beautiful introduction about how blood brings so many changes into our lives. It is written both simply and clearly, offering ways to support and hold space for our daughters at this important time of transition.

Sue Quatermass, www.goddesstemplegifts.co.uk

This is a book that mothers and daughters will enjoy reading. First Moon helps introduce the wisdom and mystery of menstruation. The words and illustrations form a bridge between the child's experience and womanhood.

Jaine Raine, www.lunawoman.com

When we're trying to bring back something precious that's been forgotten we need a guide to remind us of the way. First Moon reaches a hand out to girls as they make their journey towards womanhood, and gives their mothers the knowledge and wisdom to walk alongside their daughters.

Kim McCabe, author of *From Daughter to Woman*
www.ritesforgirls.com

I first read Anke Mai's book many years ago in a moon lodge library. Her words of wisdom are so needed in our girl's lives. The illustrations are beautiful, and I love the celebration stories from around the world. The ideas for mentors are particularly important, as all our young women need wise women mentors.

Rachael Hertogs, www.moontimes.co.uk

A nourishing guide to menarche for girls and their mothers. This book has many gems of wisdom in it that I had not come across elsewhere. I look forward to sharing it with my own daughters.

Lucy H. Pearce, author of
Reaching for the Moon and *Moon Time,*
www.womancraftpublishing.com

For Cora and Kat

Contents

Preface

I can't remember anything about my first period. My mother told me that I was 11 years old when I started. Menstruation was seen as a curse, something to hide, to put up with; not something to feel proud of and to celebrate. Boys were lucky not to have to go through it. Nobody had taught my mother or grandmother that entering womanhood was a joyous and special occasion.

I wanted this to be different for my daughters. Celebration had always played an important part in our family life and I was looking for ideas on how to mark my daughters' menarche. There was nothing in children's literature in the late 1990s that wasn't just covering the anatomy and physiology of the reproductive system. So I decided to write something myself. I took inspiration from the Native American Kinaalda ceremony and the German book *Der Mondring* by Margaret Minker.

Back then I had no idea that the small book that I wrote and self-published for my daughters and their friends would still be going strong 18 years later, or that it would find its way not only across the UK but also as far afield as classrooms in America, and into a 'Welcome to Womanhood' pack for girls in New Zealand. It has also been wonderfully affirming to find *First Moon* in an online archive of revolutionary writing.

I am delighted to see that the tides are turning and a lot has changed since 2000. There are now some excellent books available, as well as online resources. More and more women are finding ways to mark their daughters' menarche. By honouring our daughters we will also touch our inner girls, who will most likely not have had the acknowledgement they deserved.

By honouring our daughters' first moontime we will change their lives but also our own, and those of the generations that follow. This way we will create long lasting change in our society, which still has a long way to go in embracing menstruation. Let us transform shame into pride and self-respect.

May our daughters know that they are powerful.

Anke Mai
Glastonbury, December 2018.

Part One

(For Girls)

Welcome To Womanhood

Welcome to Womanhood little Sister,
Moontime is a special time,
A time to tune into your monthly cycle,
and to flow with the rhythm of the seasons.
A time to be alone and dream,
to write a poem, to paint a picture.
To treat your body to a luxurious scented bath,
to tune your mind to Nature.
To meditate by a tree, a stream,
to gaze upon a flower, a crystal,
to talk with the Moon and the Stars.
A time to dance and sing.
To share a vision with a Friend,
to light a candle for Peace.
Moontime is a special time,
a time of releasing the old,
to make way for the new.
Of releasing your Childhood,
And realising your Womanhood.
Welcome to your Moontime little Sister.

by Lorye Keats Hopper

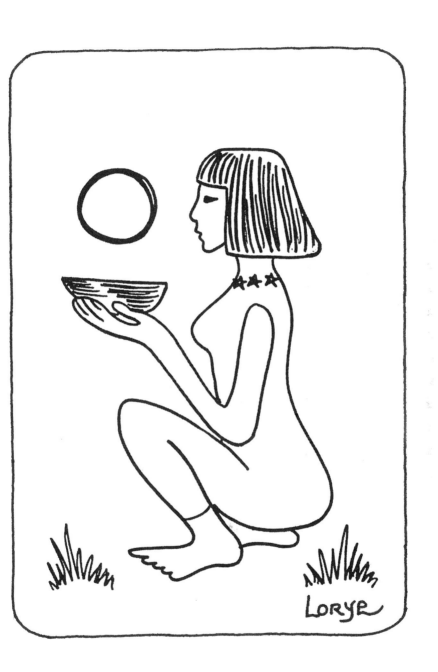

Introduction

This book is for YOU. It comes as a gift at a time in your life when your body is changing from within. You are growing from a girl into a woman, and your body is adjusting to this great change.

It is a very special time in your life, probably leaving you feeling excited, confused, scared, proud, worried, shy, curious… to mention just a few emotions. One minute you might be happy and smiling, the next minute you might feel tearful and not know why.

You will notice, when your body starts to change, when your breasts begin to feel tender and grow, when your first body hair appears.

No girl can tell in advance when she will begin to bleed, when the first day of her menstruation will come.

I will use the words 'menstruation', 'period', 'bleeding', and 'menarche' in this book. There are many other words for it like 'menses', 'days', 'flow', 'time of the month', 'being on', and 'coming on'. Some people also call it the 'curse', which is not a pleasant word. Find the word that you like best and feel most comfortable with. 'Period' is an easy word and commonly used.

You may be as young as 8 or 9 years old, or already 16 years old, when your periods start. Most likely, you will be around 11-13 years old. Every person and every body is different and special. It really doesn't matter how old you are, as long as you are well prepared for it. There are many good books available to explain all the physical changes in your body, and give you all the information you might want. A list of helpful literature is included at the end of this book under "Resources". I have also included a "Word check" for you, where you can find the meaning of words like 'menstrual cycle', 'hormones' and 'puberty'. Most of all I would recommend that you talk to your friends, mother, sister, grandmother, aunt, a teacher, school nurse or youth worker, to those women you trust and feel close to. Ask them all your questions. And find out how to use sanitary towels and tampons before your periods start. The more you know, the better you will feel about it all.

I hope that this book will help you look forward to the days when you begin to bleed. It will be your special time, when you join the circle of women. It will be a very important time in your life. Please don't let it go by unnoticed.

Once you begin to bleed every month, your body prepares itself to be able to give life, to be fertile and able to have a child of your own. However, I would strongly discourage you from getting pregnant, whilst you are still young. Although your body is ready to have a child, you are not yet ready emotionally to be a mother. A child needs a safe and secure environment to grow up in, and it is difficult to provide this as a teenager.

As you are growing into womanhood, you need to take care of your body and your newly found fertility. Look after yourself with a good diet, regular exercise and daily hygiene. Keep your body healthy and active. And most of all, love and cherish your body.

Even though you don't know when you will get your period, it is a good idea to think about it with plenty of time beforehand.

Imagine who you would like to tell about your first menstruation.

Imagine how you would like to celebrate this special time.

It will probably depend a lot on how old you are when you start to bleed.

Maybe you want to get used to it first, only tell your mum about it, or your best friend, and then think about other people too.

Maybe you don't want your periods yet, or maybe you have been waiting for a long time for them to start.

How can you make this time special in your life?

To give you some ideas, I would like to take you to some countries around the world, where girls of your age receive a special celebration. I hope that these examples will inspire you.

Enjoy your journey!

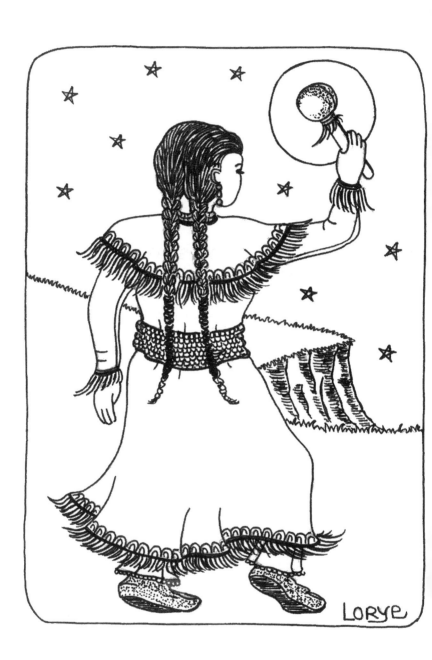

Becoming a Woman Around the World

A Journey for Girls

You might want to have a globe or atlas next to you, to look up all the countries and continents as you travel around the world.

Let us start your journey in NORTH AMERICA. Imagine YOU are a North American Indian girl, living with the Apache tribe. You have just started your period, and you are full of joy, knowing that everybody in your village will join in your special celebration.

You go to your godmother's hut and place an eagle feather at her door. With this act you are asking her to be with you during the four days of celebration. If your godmother accepts, she will teach you all you need to know about becoming a woman.

To start with, you spend some time alone in a special hut, away from other children and men. For a while you fast to cleanse your body and mind. When you are ready, your godmother teaches you that you have started to bleed because you are now fertile. This means that you can have your own children, and with this you are now a giver of life. You are very proud. Your godmother teaches you all you need to know about menstruation, fertility, sexuality and female medicine rituals. Whilst you are learning, a special dress is made for you. Your godmother also prepares you for your ceremony and teaches you a special dance. Finally, the big celebration with your whole tribe starts.

You wear your special dress and new accessories. At first you dance alone, absorbing the drumming and singing from those around you. It makes you feel strong. Now you dance the special dance of the Four Directions (you can find out more on p31). The whole community follows you in your dance. This dance symbolises your passage from birth to puberty, on to mothering, reaching maturity and wisdom in old age. It is about your growing from a baby into a girl, teenager, young adult and on into middle age and finally old age, hoping that you will be happy and well.

After the dancing finishes, cornmeal – which forms part of your daily food – and sacred plant pollen are thrown over your head. And with this you receive blessings and wishes that you may live a full life. Now it is your turn to bless the tribe, as a giver of life who will be able to have children and contribute as a woman to your village.

What a beautiful experience for you to remember and to give you strength.

Let us move on to another NORTH AMERICAN tribe, the Cheyenne. As a Cheyenne girl, you tell your mother first about the start of your menstruation. Your mother tells your father of this happy event. Meanwhile you take a cleansing bath after which your whole body is painted red. Over it you wear a special dress and you take your place of honour close to the open fire in your hut. An older woman from your community comes and sprinkles special grasses and flowers onto your fire. You lean over this sweet smelling smoke and let it cover your body. Nature's spirits are asked to protect your health and fertility.

After this smoke ritual, your father stands in the doorway of your hut and tells all the villagers that you are now a woman. You follow your grandmother into her hut, where you stay for four days and learn all about being a Cheyenne woman. After this, another smoke ritual completes your entry into womanhood.

Let us continue our journey from North America to CENTRAL AMERICA, and briefly stop in PANAMA. Here you are a girl of the Kunda Indians living on an island off the mainland. You, and several of your friends who recently started to menstruate, are having a ceremony together. You wear special clothes for this occasion, and a beautiful red, soft scarf, covered in gold embroidery and ancient symbols, is tied around your head. With this you are showing your new dignity as a woman. Your blouse also shines in strong red and gold colours, symbolising luck and fertility. Your celebration takes place in a special room, and lasts for several days.

We now leave Panama and travel down to SOUTH AMERICA, to the Aiary tribe in BRAZIL. Here your whole family and your friends gather round you after you have announced your first period. Your mother symbolically cuts off your child pigtails and gives you a new, shorter haircut. All the people present ask for a strand of your hair to keep for good luck. For a month, until your next period starts, you are only allowed to eat bread and fish. This helps to cleanse your body and mind. Once you bleed for a second time, your father gets up at sunrise to sing a special song,

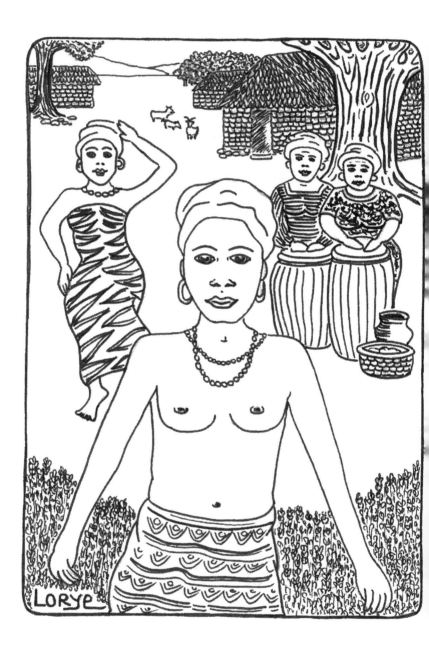

inviting everyone in your village for a feast. You can now eat as much as you like.

It is time to leave one continent behind and travel across the Atlantic Ocean to AFRICA. We arrive in NIGERIA, where you are a girl of the Tiv tribe. On the day of your first menstruation, you are seen as a fertility giver, bringing good luck. On this day, you walk across all the fields of the village, blessing the soil and helping to bring a rich harvest. During a ceremony in your honour, you receive a fertility tattoo below your navel. From now on, you proudly display this decoration to show that you are not a child any longer.

In another African country, in the CONGO, menstrual blood is celebrated as the "blood of life".

Let us move on to ZAMBIA, and visit the Luvale tribe. Here, as a young woman, you catch your first blood in a special cloth given to you by the women elders. Your grandmother buries this cloth under a holy tree to give the female power back to the earth and to ask for your protection. Once your first period has finished, you fast for a day and night. The women from your village will choose a female teacher for you. She will collect you from your hut, wrap you in a special blanket and lead you to the dance place of your ceremony. You are asked to crouch on the ground, face towards the earth, whilst the women from your tribe gather, and dance and sing around you. They dance the symbolic "death" of the girl you were, and the "rebirth" of the young woman you are now. Whilst the women dance, the men build an initiation hut for you near your mother's home. Everything for your hut has to be new, like bedding and cooking utensils. Once the hut is finished, the women lead you in a procession to your new home. A fire is lit in your hut, and your chosen teacher stays with you, whilst the community continues to dance, sing and celebrate.

In the following months, you have to learn a lot about:

○   the phases of the moon

○   recognising, collecting and preparing medicinal herbs

○   sexuality, contraception, pregnancy and childbirth

○   tending your hut fire, fishing, food gathering and cooking

○   storytelling

○   a special dance movement to prepare you for lovemaking and childbirth.

You are also expected to have inner peace and strength, and work hard in your community. Once your learning phase is complete, you will be given another celebration during the next full moon. You are washed by the women of your village, your hair is plaited and your body is covered in vegetable oil and red earth. You are allowed to join in the women's dance for the first time. You are very proud and happy.

In another African country, ZIMBABWE, you can take on a new name once you have started to menstruate.

Let us leave the African continent behind and travel across the Indian Ocean to ASIA. Imagine that you are a girl living in SRI LANKA. Here, on the first day of your menses a horoscope of the stars and planets is drawn up to give your family information about your future years of marriage. Afterwards you have a ritual bath. You leave your girlhood behind and step out of the bath as a young woman. You dress all in white, the colour of initiation. Your family gives you a celebration, during which you receive many gifts and wishes of good luck.

If you lived in CAMBODIA your parents would plant a banana tree at the time of your first menstruation. The fruit of this tree would be for you alone to harvest and eat.

In JAPAN a party would be held for all your friends and relatives. The festive table would be decorated with red flowers, candied red apples and red coloured rice.

After this brief visit to Asia we move on to AUSTRALIA. Imagine yourself now as an Aboriginal girl. Here it is a custom that, once you have started to menstruate, your mother and grandmother build a hut for you. You will spend a few days on your own in it, resting, meditating and receiving messages in your dreams. This will make you feel stronger inside, as you are now ready to start life as a woman. All the women of your village will gather for a celebration. They will dance and sing, and give thanks for the female power that lives within you. They will give thanks for the physical changes of your growing body, which now can bear and feed children, like Mother Earth gives birth to plants, animals and humans, and provides for them.

To complete our journey, let us travel across the PACIFIC OCEAN back to NORTH AMERICA, where we started. Our last country is CANADA where I would like you to join the Nootka tribe. All the children in this community learn to swim from an early age. Girls are expected to show their strength, courage and power by swimming a long distance. You, and other young women who have just started their period, go out to sea in a specially decorated boat. You jump into the water and swim back to the shore, encouraged by the cheers from the people rowing your

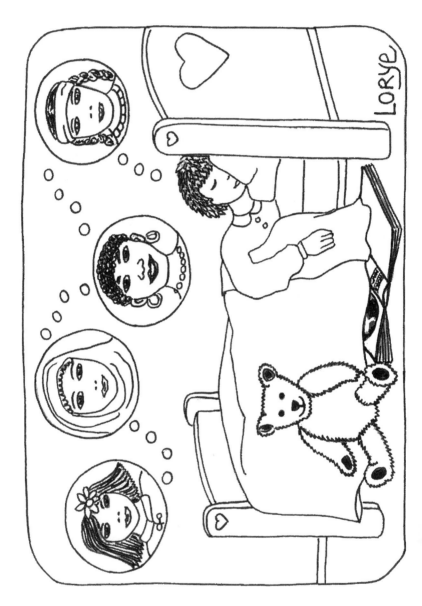

boat. They stay close to you. On the beach, a big welcome by all your family and friends awaits you, followed by an all-night party.

You have come to the end of your journey around the world, and it is time to return to your own country.

Did you enjoy your travels?
Did you learn from all these traditions?
Do you feel inspired to start looking at your own celebration?

Even if we do not live in tribal communities, we can find ideas and inspirations in these traditions. Some of the ceremonies I have described are still practised today, whilst others are no longer followed. All of the mentioned traditions have a lot in common, and I would like to have a closer look at these elements in the next chapter.

Celebration – Planning Your Special Day

Ideas for mothers and daughters to discuss together

The word 'celebrate' comes from the ancient Greek *melpo* meaning 'to sing, to dance, to praise'.[i]

By deciding to celebrate your first menstruation, you are making a statement to the world that YOU matter. That you are important and that this celebration marks an important passage in your life. Let this event nurture you and help to make you feel strong and good about yourself.

As you don't know when your periods will start, it is a good idea to think about it beforehand and to have some plans and preparations ready. It is YOUR day, and you can choose to spend this day in the way that you want. Of course you will need the agreement and support of your family or carer.

Most likely, you don't know yet how you will feel and what you will want to do. You don't have to do anything at all. Just going through this big transition may be enough in itself for you.

You will probably tell your mum about it first. Maybe you will talk to your best friend about it too. You might want some time to yourself. Maybe you will feel tired and achy and not like any company at all. Your period might start when you are still quite young, and you might feel like waiting for a celebration until you are a bit older, when some of your friends are menstruating too. You could decide to have a party or day out together. Or you might have lots of plans ready and want a celebration as soon as possible.

It is up to you and your family, to make this time special. If you decide to have a celebration/party/ceremony/gathering, think about who you would want to invite. Family? Friends? Girls and women only? How do you feel about telling your brother, father, uncle or grandfather?

If you want a special celebration, think about what would make you feel good and special.

Go through the list of options in this chapter. Take your time, and talk to your mother, carer and also your friends about it. Maybe you can come up with your own ideas.

Decide if you want to be involved in planning and preparing your celebration, or if you would rather have a surprise present or outing. Talk to your family to see what is actually realistic for your situation, including money matters.

And if you are reading this book as a young woman or adult and already have your periods, but feel that you have missed out on a celebration, don't worry. Invite your women friends, use your imagination and give yourself a special day.

If we refer to your "Journey around the world", we will see that all these celebrations have a lot in common.

Time Alone

In many cultures a special hut is built for the newly menstruating girl. She spends some time away from the rest of the community. Here she finds the space to go inward,

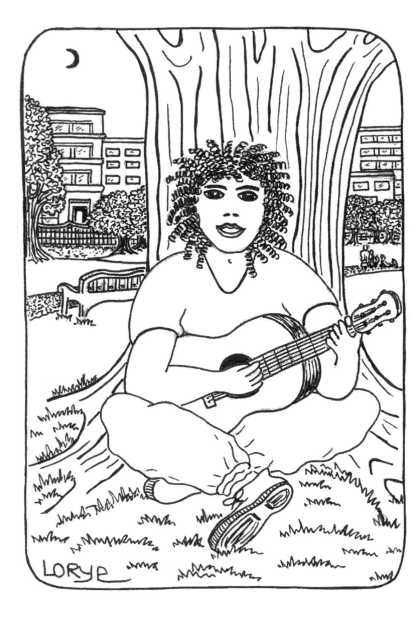

LORYE

to find her inner strength and knowledge. Often she is accompanied by an older woman.

During pre-puberty and puberty your body is in great transition. You are changing, growing from a girl into a woman. Your hormones and emotions may leave you feeling tired and vulnerable.

During 'Time Alone' you can find your inner peace and strength again. You can be with yourself and adjust to your inner and outer changes. 'Time Alone' can happen in many different ways. Here are some options. See if you like the sound of them. Wherever you live, you can find a way to be on your own for a while, if it is important to you.

○ You could choose to have a day/night/weekend away from your normal routine. Stay with a relative or friend who is willing to look after you, and who is willing to respect your need for quiet space.

○ You could put up a tent in your garden, or if you are lucky enough, in a field or woodland near your home. Spend a night by yourself. Ask your siblings to leave you alone. You may want to ask someone to keep guard nearby, especially in a woodland or field, to make sure you are safe.

○ You could find your own special tree and sit under it, in your garden, park or woodland nearby. Get to know your tree and follow your dreams under it.

○ Lie in the grass and look up at the sky.

○ Go for a bike ride.

○ Take your dog for a walk.

○ Hire a rowing boat in the park.

o   Take a bath with your favourite bubbles.

o   Go to your room and listen to some music.

o   Write a daily journal.

Fasting

Not eating food for a day or longer, or only eating certain foods, is a way to cleanse your body and soul. With this you are honouring the transition that your body is going through. However, this is not something to do or decide on your own. If you are deciding on a more spiritual ceremony, you could have a cleansing day beforehand of eating only fruit and drinking plenty of water. You will need your parents' or guardians' agreement.

Bathing

Another way to cleanse your body, and leave the 'old you' behind, is by taking a ritual bath. You could make it a part of your ceremony or celebration. Or you could simply just enjoy this special bath, after you started bleeding for the first time. Use your favourite bath foam, bath oil and scatter scented herbs or flowers onto the water. Light candles, if you are allowed, and play some nice music. Enjoy! It is a lovely way to look after your body.

What will you do after your special bath?
Celebrate with your family and friends?
Go out for a meal with your mum?
Go camping for the night with your dad?
Go to bed for some time alone?

Clothes

Would you enjoy wearing special clothes as part of your celebration?

Do you remember the celebration colours from our "Journey around the world"? They were white, red and gold: white for purity, red for your menstrual blood and gold for special occasions. Do you like any of these colours? Do you know which ones suit you?

Would you like to wear clothes in any of these colours for your special day? You could have a look at your own clothes, or borrow some from your sister or friend. Maybe your family can afford to buy you a new outfit for this occasion.

A red scarf is a lovely present at this time. You could wear it each month when you are bleeding. Maybe your mum, sister, granny or aunt would like to embroider onto it.

Wear whatever makes you feel good.

Hair / Make-up / Perfume

Do you like your hair? This might be a good time in your life to have a change of style.

Do you like using make-up, or are you not sure about it? Ask your mum or friend for advice. Would an appointment with a beautician be a way to celebrate for you? Or buying your first own make-up?

Would you like to try out some perfume? Maybe you could choose your own bottle. Ask your mum or carer to help you.

Maybe you know all about make-up already and it is nothing special any longer. Or maybe you don't like the idea of make-up at all.

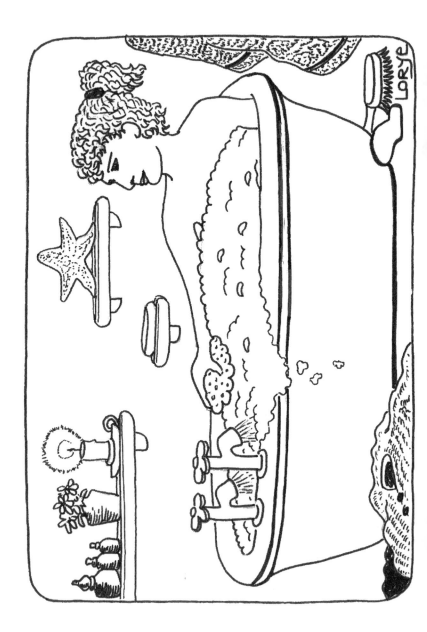

Does body painting appeal to you? You could invite your friends and paint your body red, or try out natural plant and earth pigments. Ask an adult to help you with this. Go for a walk together and try to find natural colouring materials, like clay and plants.

Have fun, whatever you do.

Jewellery

This is an occasion to receive your own special jewellery. Maybe you will be given a piece of family jewellery, a necklace, a bracelet or a ring. Or maybe you would like to go out with your mother or family and choose a necklace or ring to mark the day that you started to menstruate. Maybe you don't like the idea of a party or celebration with your family. You want to do something private and special in a different way. It also doesn't need to cost a lot of money. You could choose a small ring with a red stone or maybe a moon-design. A ring would be a lovely way to remember this time which only comes once in your life.

If you are interested in stones and crystals, you could choose the one which has the most meaning to you. And it doesn't need to be red. Or you could choose a ring with a moon on it, as a symbol of your closeness to nature and its changing cycles, just like your own now. You could choose a ring with your star sign, or one with a woman's symbol on it.

You could ask for the date of your first menstruation to be engraved into the ring or other piece of jewellery. This would make it even more special.

Flowers

Most celebrations and ceremonies include the use of flowers. Do you like flowers? If you do, I hope you will have lots of flowers around you at this special time. Maybe your mum or dad will pick or buy you flowers when you start to menstruate to congratulate you on your way to becoming a woman. You could wear a flower crown or garland for your celebration. Or scatter pink and red flower petals in your bath. Use flowers to decorate your dinner table or party room.

Maybe you would like to plant a small tree or scented rosebush in your garden, to mark this special day. You could choose a tree with red fruit, like cherries or apples, which are only yours to harvest and eat.

Getting up-to-date

This is also a good time in your life to get up-to-date. Maybe you have outgrown some of your toys, books and clothes. Maybe you would like to change the wallpaper or paint colour in your room. Could you help your parents redecorate?

And what about your name? Are people calling you by your childhood nickname? Do you still like this? Or would you like to be called by your real name instead now?

Look at your life and see where an outer change might be needed to match your transition from a girl into a woman. It is good to talk to your parents about this.

I hope that the ideas above have inspired you to think about your own celebration. Of course you can't expect to do all of this. Think about what appeals to you most:

- Do you want a quiet celebration? A meal out? A day out? A special present?

- Do you want a celebration with family and/or friends? A meal at home with all your family? A party with your friends?

- Do you want a spiritual ceremony? A ritual and blessing? An evening of dance, drumming and storytelling?

Think about who you would like to invite.
Think about where you would like to meet.
Think about food, room decorations, music, invitations etc.
Think about what you would like to wear.
Ask someone to help you with all the preparations.

And a note for mothers:

If your daughter is old enough and wants to be actively involved in the preparations of her celebration, let her do her share. However, you might decide that you want to do most of it for her, after you have discussed her options with her.

Or maybe you decide that a 'gathering' is not a good idea at this time. You might like to celebrate in a very different way: quieter or more personal for just the two of you.

Or you might want to give her a surprise present, which also doesn't have to cost a lot. You could ask the female members of your family to join in a craft project. You could make a special patchwork quilt between you, or an embroidery together, or a photo album of all the female family members. You could make her a necklace with beads given by all family members, or write a collection of poems for her. Use your imagination and creativity.

Or you might feel drawn to do some travelling with your daughter. This would be a good time to take her to one of the sacred sites of the Goddess, for example Glastonbury.

Project / Practical task

Your daughter might be into her teens by the time her periods start. She no longer sees herself as a child and wants society to recognise that she is growing and changing on all levels. She begins to understand her increased responsibility towards society, and she is aware that she is walking on stepping stones towards full adulthood. As she is growing physically and mentally, she could mark the beginning of menstruation with a special project or task. She could set herself a challenge, which will stretch her, test her abilities, or affirm her responsibilities towards others and the planet we live on.

You could talk to her about her future role as an adult, and about practical ideas to mark this transition.

Your daughter could set herself a physical task, which will test her limits: a long distance run, taking part in a riding competition, climbing a mountain, cycling or swimming further than she has done so far. She could find sponsors for this task, and prove her strength and power, as well as collect money for a charity.

If she is not interested in sport, she could set herself a practical task: volunteering in an ecological project, joining in local community activities like visiting ill children in hospital or helping in an old people's home.

The project or task could be followed by a ceremony or celebration with family and friends. Depending on the age of your daughter, this could be more of a Coming of Age

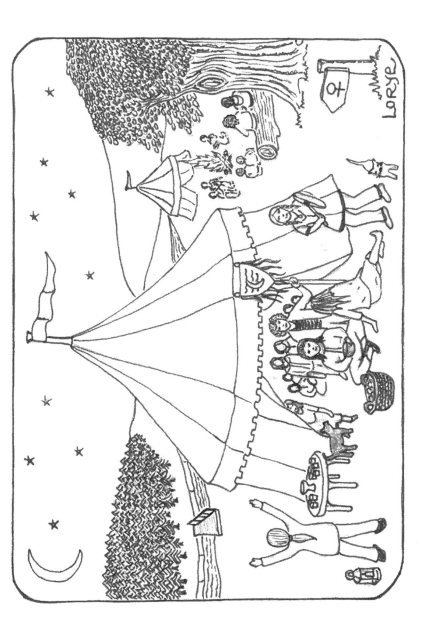

celebration, welcoming and honouring her as a woman.

It is very appropriate for a young woman at this stage in her life to choose a mentor. Parents are normally the least appropriate people to guide young people through initiation. Teenagers have to break away from the influence of their parents and find their own way in the world. However, adults need to provide structure, boundaries and a safe environment for young people who want to test their abilities and limits. In our society teenagers often try to initiate themselves by danger-seeking activities such as taking drugs or joyriding. Initiation is not something young people can do for themselves, but something through which they must be guided by an adult.

Talk to your daughter, look at her needs and set up an appropriate challenge for her, which she can complete.

Spiritual Ceremony

Puberty rites, or Coming of Age ceremonies are usually performed with only women present. However, the male members of your family should also be included in some part of the ceremony. Puberty ceremonies are usually held soon after the first menstruation, often during the new moon following the menstruation. Or they take place during a special time of the year, such as the spring, when the plants begin to bloom, a time when May Day celebrations and Fertility Rites are traditionally held. Often a group of girls hold a ceremony together at this time of the year.

Depending on your daughter's age and your family circumstances, the ceremony can be as simple or as elaborate as you wish. You could hold a private, family only, blessing followed by a party for all her friends.

The ceremony could include the use of candles, incense, chants, poems, prayers, ceremonial objects etc.

You might want to refer to the four directions in your special menstruation ceremony. Many Native American tribes relate the 'Four Directions' to the four stages of life a woman moves through.

North to East	The first quadrant on the Native American medicine wheel refers to ages 0 – 13, birth to puberty. The childhood and learning 'everything' period.
East to South	The second quadrant, refers to the 'mothering' period. From menstruation to first child, from nurturing your own family to also being actively involved in the community.
South to West	The third quadrant is the period of maturity. After being concerned about your own family and community, the relationship to the larger world now becomes important. The time of grandchildren begins and of being a mentor to young women. Menopause marks the transition from the third into the fourth quadrant.
West to North	The fourth quadrant refers to the period of the 'True Self'. It is you and the Great Mystery, the meaning of life and moving towards your own death.

In the Apache tradition, when a young girl comes of age and begins to bleed, she is welcomed into womanhood by her entire tribe. She learns the steps of the 'Sunrise Dance' and 'Changing Woman', the proud giver of all life. First the girl dances alone, then the entire community joins in. The young girl runs in the four directions, whilst the community runs behind her. They do this to express their desire that the girl live through the four stages of life. The dancing is followed by the tribe blessing the girl, and in return, the girl, acting as 'Changing Woman', blessing the tribe. Both dancing and also fasting continue for four days.[ii]

The book *Women's Medicine Ways: Cross-Cultural Rites of Passage,* by Marcia Starck contains a chapter on Puberty Ceremonies, as well as many beautiful chants, which you might like to include in your ceremony.

Red Party

If your daughter simply wants to have some fun with her friends, you could suggest the idea of a Red Party.

In many cultures red is the colour of joy and fertility. Red is also the colour of royalty, symbolising strength and power. Red is the warmest of all colours. In some cultures, girls are covered in red paint once they start bleeding, or they wear a red headscarf or receive a red scarf, which they wear with pride from then on, as a symbol of their womanhood. And red is also the colour of the menstrual blood.

You could plan a Red Party for her celebration. Use the colour red to decorate your kitchen or dining room: red flowers, scarves, ribbons, red lanterns or balloons and red candles will look good. Maybe your daughter would like to wear red, and her guests could be asked to wear some red too.

Next, think about which red foods or drinks you could offer. Have some fun together with your daughter.

Foods	Red fruits include strawberries, raspberries, redcurrants, cherries, apples, melon, red oranges, and also pomegranates, an ancient symbol of female fertility. You could make a big bowl of red fruit salad. Or you could use red fruit in the form of ice cream, sorbet, yogurt, jam or fruit juice. Red vegetables include tomatoes, peppers, beetroot, cabbage, radishes, some varieties of lettuce leaves, and also red onions. Again you could make a red salad, or a soup, stuff red peppers or make a pizza with red toppings. Here you could include red meat like pepperami slices. You could also use red pasta.
Drinks	Red drinks include fruit juices, vegetable juices, herbal teas or maybe a first taste of red wine.

You could also hard boil eggs, as a symbol of your daughter's new fertility. She could paint them red with her friends, or colour them with beetroot juice.

Maybe your daughter would enjoy writing out a menu in advance, again in red, and make name cards for the table.

The meal could be followed by some storytelling, a shared craft activity or dancing.

Moontime

Did you know that your periods and the moon are closely related? That some women called their periods 'moontime' in the past? The words 'menstruate' and 'menses' come from the Latin *mensis*, which means 'month'. An average menstrual cycle lasts as long as it takes the moon to circle around the earth, 29.5 days. Many cultures have noticed that the moon's phases, from new moon to full moon, and the woman's menstrual cycle are closely linked.

Chinese women started a moon calendar 3000 years ago, writing down 28 'houses' through which the moon passed. Every woman of the Mayan culture in Central America knew that the Great Mayan Calendar had first been based on the women's menstrual cycle. The Romans also calculated their time – a calendar month – on the basis of menstruation.

The moon usually is thought of as female, and the sun as male. Stories are told that, in the past, all the women of some communities would menstruate at the same time of the month, usually during new moon, whilst the full moon is the time for greatest fertility and ovulation - the time to conceive a child. Also, all over the world, many women give birth during full moon. In our modern society, women have lost touch with the moon cycle. It is now time to reclaim this connection.

You could have a look at your own menstrual cycle and the moon phases. You can buy moon charts and calendars, and a lot of ordinary diaries and calendars tell you when it is full moon or new moon.

It is a good idea to mark your own menstrual cycle on a calendar each month. Write down the days and dates of your period. Note the length of your cycle. You could also keep a personal mood chart, writing down how your cycle affects your feelings. Some days you might feel great, whilst on others you might feel more tearful and low in energy.

When you first start your periods, your cycle might still be quite irregular. The length of your cycle is the number of days between the start of one period and the next. It may be as short as 21 days or as long as 35 days, or anything in between. The length of your period - the number of days that you bleed - will also vary from woman to woman. Some days may be lighter and you bleed less, and some days heavier, with more blood loss. Ask your mum, sister or friend to help you find your own way of recording your periods and see where your cycle is in relation to the moon cycle.

If you like the moon and feel close to it, you could hold your celebration at new moon. Or you could ask for a special moon present to mark the beginning of your periods, maybe a ring, necklace or earrings with the moon symbol. You could also include the moon in your party. There are many moon decorations available, like candles, cards, lanterns, pictures etc. You could ask for a moon story to be told, or make up a moon dance. Many songs also talk about the moon. Or you could simply go for a quiet moon walk and let the moon speak to you.[iii]

Painful Periods

Information for girls and their guardians

Your periods will probably be irregular to start with; weeks, even months, may go by before your next period arrives.

You may also experience pain with your periods. Quite often a pulling sensation around your stomach, womb and lower back may tell you that another period is starting.

If you do get painful periods you could try:

○ Hugging a hot-water bottle against your tummy.

○ Taking a hot bath. You could try adding a few drops of relaxing oils like lavender or chamomile.

○ Massaging your stomach and lower back. You could add a few drops of essential oils with a relaxing effect to some base oil like almond or coconut. Try marjoram, lavender or chamomile first. Clary sage, myrrh and sage will reduce pain, but also increase your blood flow. Avoid these oils if your periods are heavy and, especially, if you are pregnant. Geranium and rose will help with heavy periods; rose will also help with irregular cycles. You can find out more about these oils in books on aromatherapy. Essential oils are available at chemists, health and wholefood shops, or by mail-order. Check with an adult that they are safe to use for you.

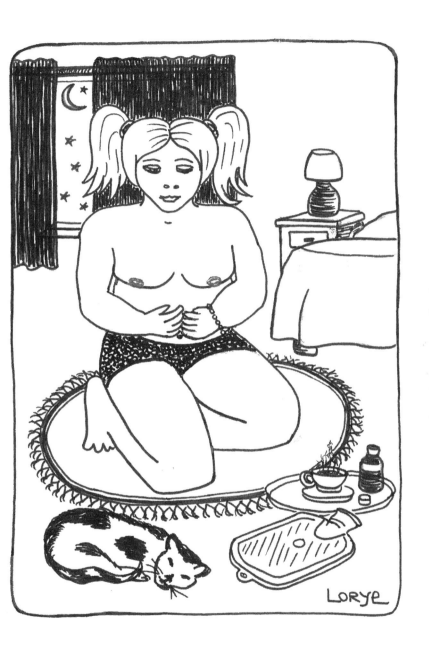

- Try to relax, curl up with a good book, breathe deeply, maybe learn some yoga exercises to help with painful periods.

- Make sure you eat well, especially fresh fruit and vegetables, and drink plenty of water.

- Exercise if you can. You might not feel like it, but you will feel better for it afterwards. Cycle, take the dog for a walk, dance to your favourite music, try some exercises to strengthen your stomach and pelvic muscles.

- Instead of taking a painkiller, try drinking some herbal teas.

- Be nice to yourself!

Herbs

You can grow your own, buy them in dried form in your local health food shop, or mail-order them from herbal suppliers. There are lots of good books available on herbs, providing all the information you will need.

The most commonly used herbs for painful periods are:

Cramp Bark (Viburnum opulus)

The bark is collected in April and May, cut into pieces and dried. It is a bitter herb to take, but has a relaxing effect on the uterus.

Black Haw (Viburnum prunifolium)

The bark from the roots and the trunk is collected in the autumn. The bark from the branches is collected in the spring and summer. Black Haw is closely related to Cramp

Bark; it is another powerful relaxant to the uterus that is commonly used for painful periods.

Black Haw combines well with Jamaican Dogwood (*Piscidia erythrina*) for painful periods.

Black Cohosh (Cimicifuga racemosa)

The root is collected in the autumn, cut and dried. Another bitter herb with a powerful relaxing action on the uterus, it also balances the female hormones.

Yarrow (Achillea millefolium)

The whole of the plant above ground is collected when it flowers between June and September. It is especially used for heavy bleeding.

Lady's Mantle (Alchemilla vulgaris)

The leaves and stems are collected in July and August. Lady's Mantle will help with period pains, also with excessive bleeding.

Motherwort (Leonurus cardiaca)

The stalks are collected at the time of flowering, between June and September.

Motherwort helps with menstrual and uterine conditions. It is especially used for delayed or suppressed menstruation, often associated with tension and anxiety. It is a useful tonic for menopausal changes. It is also excellent for the heart.

There are many other herbs that can help with your menstrual cycle. Go to the local library or bookshop to find out more about healing plants.

To use any of these, pour a cup of boiling water onto 1-2 teaspoons of the dried herb, and leave it to infuse for 10-15 minutes. Strain, and drink one cupful three times a day.

Please ask an adult to help you with the preparation of herbal teas. If you don't like the taste, add some sweetener like honey. If you still don't like it, try taking the herbs as a tincture. I am not a qualified health practitioner. If you do have ongoing problems with your periods, I recommend contacting the National Institute of Medical Herbalists (if you live in the UK) to find a qualified herbalist near you.

www.nimh.org.uk

Cherish Your Body

As your body grows from girl to woman, you will notice many changes. It is much easier to look at your breasts, your widening hips, your pubic hair, and your armpits, than it is to look at your vagina. I would encourage you to get a small handheld mirror, and to find somewhere private like your bedroom or bathroom and have a look at your vagina. You might feel embarrassed doing this, but be assured that this is perfectly normal and necessary for you to learn about your body. It will help you feel good about being a woman.

A lot of teenage girls don't like parts of their bodies, and are very critical about themselves. There is a lot of pressure on girls and women to look a certain way. Try to remember that everybody is different and special. Girls can help each other to feel good about the way they look. Treat your body gently and make sure that others treat it gently, too. This is your precious body.

You will probably have mixed feelings about the idea of touching and kissing another person. There is no need to rush into it. Your sexual awakening will unfold gradually over the years, and you will have the rest of your life to explore, express, and enjoy your sexuality. Many people find it embarrassing to talk about sex openly and honestly. But there is no need to feel embarrassed or ashamed, sex is a natural part of our lives. Get to know and like your body.

Remember that your body is yours alone. Don't let anyone touch it in a way that doesn't feel right. Trust your feelings and follow them. Don't do anything that you don't want to do. And don't let anyone put you under pressure to act against your will. It is your body and you are in charge of it. Nobody else is. Be gentle and loving with yourself. Always.

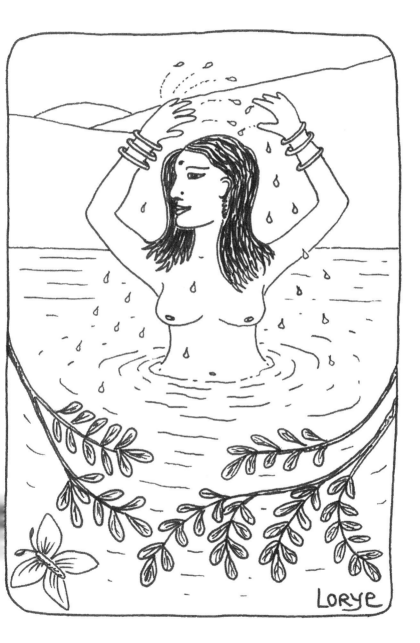

LORYE

Contributions (part one)

My First Blood Story

I had been given the job of returning a horse from its paddock to a field, a distance of only about half a mile. It was a fluke that I had been asked to do it. I was eleven years old and no-one knew that I felt that it was the most exciting thing that I had ever been asked to do. The rather large horse had a bridle but no saddle, so I rather nervously clambered onto its back, without any previous riding experience but with a genuine feeling of ancient confidence. The horse knew exactly what was happening. It was the end of a hard day's work and pastures were much greener in the field that she knew she was heading to, so she just took off at full gallop. The most amazing feelings occurred as I realised my body could easily respond to the movement of the horse without any fear of falling off.

By the time we got there (which didn't take very long!), I was absolutely exhilarated. When I got off, I thought that I had wet myself with excitement... I asked my companion, who was riding the other horse, to go on without me, and I found a suitable bush where I examined myself. I found that I had begun to bleed for the very first time. For this to have happened during one of the most exciting and memorable moments of my life was the most wonderful thing and I felt that the experience was a sign of the true gift of life.

It was a double celebration for me, the first was that I was now a woman and the second was that to become so while fulfilling one of my wildest dreams left me feeling greatly honoured; not, funnily enough, by my family or society, but by life itself.

And the last thing I would like to say to any young girl is that where society, school or family seem to fail you, you can be certain that your life is celebrated and loved by an unseen Lover that reveals itself to whatever degree you allow it to.

Sandra Bruce

Menarche

A few months after my thirteenth birthday I began to bleed. From the moment of my first blood I had an awareness of my body that was different; it felt like a secret, a claim and a threshold.

Though I come from a community of spiritual people reclaiming traditions and ceremony I was one of the first of my age group to receive a full menarche celebration. My mum spent a long time researching and designing the most beautiful and perfect day for me.

I didn't know what would happen until the day and I felt so shy and proud at the same time.

I invited women and girls that were closest to me in my life.

In preparation I went with my Goddess mother to buy something red that I would love to wear as I was welcomed into womanhood in the ceremony.

A friend decorated a wooden box with moons and red velvet to be my moon box that would be filled with treasures to open at my next moontime.

My mum built a red tent space in the garden that was bright and sumptuous.

It was a day that was really about me and my becoming, who I am and what kind woman I wanted to be. It was such an honouring, initiation and blessing.

After shedding and letting go of my white cloak of maidenhood I was crowned in flowers, invited into the circle of women and heard their experiences, stories and words of wisdom.

I was showered in gifts and recognition, red roses, poems and ribbons.

My grandmother wrote me songs that we sang together and that have since been part of many menarches.

I danced in the sun with my feet on the earth and slept under the stars nestled beside my sisters.

It had all the elements of a party with the feasting, gifts and pretty dresses but also had the depth of a ceremony with the tears and laughter, focus and prayer. It was special and profound.

The attention and love that was given to me poured into my bones and stayed there, nourishing me and feeding me.

It has been 10 years and I still remember that day with huge gratitude. It is still one of my best memories of my life so far.

If I have daughters I want to give them a menarche like mine.

Physically I have a had a difficult journey with my moontime. The support and guidance I received that day helped me to remember to stay connected to my body and to listen to myself and I give thanks for how much my moontime has taught me to look after myself, that lesson is invaluable.

Gabrielle O'Connell

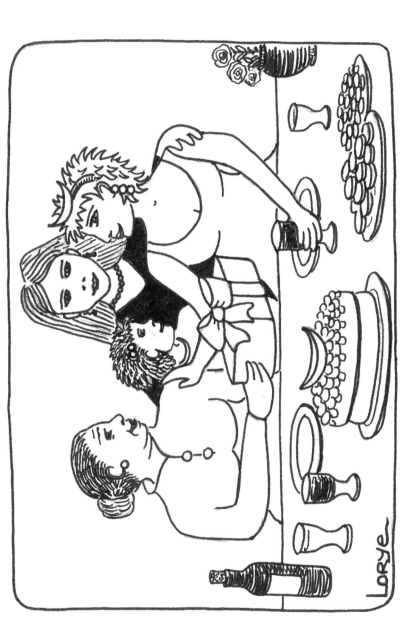

Lorye

Menarchy

I started bleeding when I was fourteen, and even though I grew up in a tradition that was very open and celebrated women's first blood, I did not have my Menarchy until I was sixteen. Mostly this was because I was scared and embarrassed by what was happening to my body. Even though all of my family and friends were open about periods, I still felt that it was something shameful.

After some time I became more comfortable with it. I accepted it and I also recognised that my embarrassment was normal, especially in the society we live in today. I no longer felt that my period was a frightening thing beyond my control and neither did I feel bad about my initial embarrassment, I was ready to celebrate this step into womanhood.

And so I did. I invited a group of women who are important to me and have played a part in my life. Young women and older women, mothers and daughter and sisters. We sat in circle and they told me about their own experiences and shared wisdom and knowledge that they had discovered throughout their lives.

They sang to me, gave me gifts and welcomed me into womanhood. During the course of the ceremony a box had been filled with gifts, and words of love, I could open it when I bled next and I would receive all the support that this circle of women had woven. At the end of it we shared a huge feast of delicious foods: chocolate and cake and juicy fruits.

I am glad that I waited until I felt that I was ready to celebrate my bleeding and I am glad that I did not feel that too much time had passed and not have a Menarchy. It was an important ceremony for me to have and I think that it is important for all young women to experience something similar.

Avena Rawnsley

Vision Quest

When I was 16 I did a Vision Quest to mark my transition into womanhood. I had a mentor, who helped me prepare for it. We met about once a month, and I would prepare a meal in exchange for her teaching. The Vision Quest itself involved camping in nature by myself for two nights. It was a time to be alone. A time to journey. To test oneself. To find out who you were and who you wanted to be. A circle of women stayed nearby, encouraging me in spirit and singing to me during the night. When the Vision Quest was over they welcomed me into the circle of womanhood, and each gave me a gift. I sat at the head of the circle, dressed in new clothes I had been asked by the mentor to sew myself.

It took a long time for me to feel the full effect of the Vision Quest or want to speak about it to others, as it was such a personal journey. But I think it helped give me a confidence and a certainty deep within me of my own self. I then had that certainty to draw on as I moved into womanhood, as I trod the uncertain path of life. However you chose to do it, undertaking an experience that challenges you, especially through being in nature, will help you learn who you are.

Cora Mia

Word-check

Coming of age	The time when a child turns into an adult.
Contraception	Birth control or Family Planning, are all names given to the different ways of stopping a woman from getting pregnant during sex. Contraceptives like using a condom, or taking the Pill, stop you having a baby.
Fertility	Being fertile, the time during your menstrual cycle when you are most likely to get pregnant. Being able to have children.
Hormones	These are natural chemicals that your body produces. They cause the changes in your body during puberty.
Hygiene	Personal hygiene, looking after your growing body and keeping it clean.

Initiation	Celebrating the beginning of a different stage in your life, introducing something new. Starting school, starting college or work, getting married, starting a family. Initiation rituals often mark the change from a child to an adult.
Menopause	When your periods stop, usually when you are around fifty years old.
Menstrual cycle	The time from the beginning of one period to the beginning of the next.
Puberty	The time when your body starts to change from a girl's to a woman's; pre-puberty means before this change starts.
Rites of passage	A major turning point in your life. For girls and women those include your first period, giving birth to a child, stopping your periods when you are older.
Ritual	A special ceremony/event for example, one to welcome a new baby, to mark the change from a child to an adult, to celebrate a marriage or to say good-bye to a person who has died.

Sanitary towels	Soak up the blood from your period, as it leaves your body. Sanitary towels stick to the inside of your underpants. You can also use washable sanitary towels or pads. They come in lovely colours and patterns, and are made from soft cotton. You fasten them to your underpants with poppers. Washable pads and panty liners are chemical free, save you a lot of money over time as you can re-use them. They are kind to your body, kind to your purse, and kind to the environment. Washable pads are used by women of all ages.
Spotting	Losing a few drops/spots of blood. Light bleeding.
Tampons	Fit inside your vagina and absorb the blood from your periods before it leaves your body. Some women prefer using washable sponges made of natural fibre. Sponges can be re-used and contain no harmful chemicals. They fit inside your vagina like tampons. Some older girls and women also use mooncups. These are small rubber cups that collect the blood before it enters your vagina, and can be washed out and used again.

I have probably only mentioned a few of the words that you don't understand. Ask a friend, older sister, mother or other adult to explain the other words to you.

Part Two

(For Mothers and other Guardians)

Introduction

Today, in Western cultures, the onset of menstruation is usually not honoured by ceremony or ritual.

Our daughters may be better informed and have a wide choice of sanitary products available, however, they are still affected by the negative attitude towards menstruation. It is still largely a shameful subject, often talked about in secret, and many women continue to see the monthly bleeding as a 'curse'.

I think the time has come to celebrate ourselves and our daughters; to increase our own, and our daughters' self-esteem, and to prepare them well for the onset of menstruation. We should start at an early age, and hopefully our daughter's first bleeding will be anticipated with pride and joy.

It should also be understood and respected by all persons in her life, including her father and brothers if she has them.

Today, some girls start menstruation as young as 8 or 9 years old. Preparation has to begin early, depending on the girl's interest and willingness to talk about her changing body.

It is also important to remember that the year before the onset of menstruation is usually one of heightened sensitivity and emotionality, due to hormonal changes.

Your daughter may be 9, 11 or 16 years old, when she begins to bleed. Therefore it is important to find the right way of celebration, appropriate for her age; as well as for your financial and family circumstances, and religious beliefs.

This book will give you ideas and help with the decision.

May you and the girls in your life enjoy reading "First Moon" and feel inspired to create your own celebration!

Your daughter will gradually change and grow, on her way to becoming a woman. 'First blood' is a very important time in this process and ceremony and ritual are spiritual ways to help young women across the threshold to adult-hood.

Be prepared to also feel sadness, as well as joy, as your daughter is gradually leaving childhood behind.

I wish you well on your journey together.

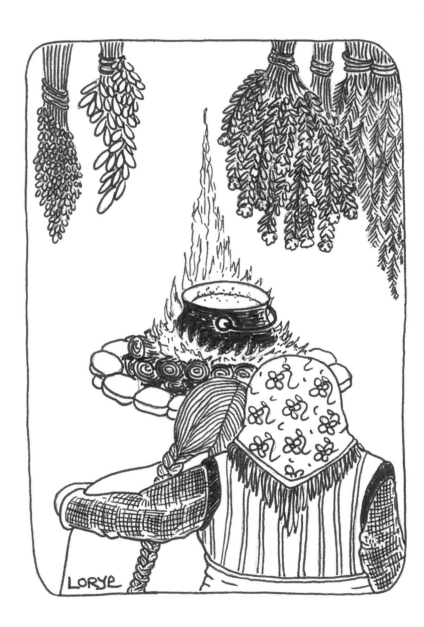

Wise Woman

In many cultures, a 'Wise Woman', an older woman, is chosen as a mentor for the young woman who has just started to menstruate. The mentor acts as a guide, as a teacher and companion to the younger woman. She gives advice and help, and traditionally would prepare the newly menstruating girl for her role as a woman.

The Wise Woman would not be the mother of the girl. Sometimes the grandmother acts as a mentor, or the women of the girl's community choose a suitable guide.

I think the time has come to reclaim this tradition of teaching and, especially, WELCOMING our daughters into womanhood.

As our daughters grow into women and take their first steps into society, they will need to 'turn away' from their families. During the adolescent years, our daughters will begin their journey to find themselves and their own position in the world. During this transition stage, our daughters will need teachers, guides, advisors, and companions. A mentor can take some weight and responsibility off our shoulders, as mothers, and act as a companion to us as well.

A mother's role will still be very important, but our daughters will also need someone else to turn to, to talk to about becoming a woman. From menstruation to sexuality, body image, and first love, someone they can trust, and someone who will not go and immediately tell us all the details. Our daughters will need a woman who acts like an older friend, and someone who shows by example how good it feels to be a woman.

A mentor acts as an independent advisor and companion, who is not involved in the mother-daughter dynamic as well as a representative of the outside world, into which the girl is taking her own independent steps.

Who could act as a mentor in our society and how would you go about choosing the right woman?

Talk to your daughter and see if you both think that it is a good idea to find a mentor for her. Find someone close by, who your daughter can meet with and talk to on a regular basis. Find someone you both like and especially someone you can both trust. It could be:

○ an aunt

○ a grandmother

○ a godmother

○ a close female friend of your family

○ a teacher

○ a youth worker

○ a work colleague

○ a much-valued neighbour

Being a mentor is a big responsibility and a commitment over several years. Your chosen 'Wise Woman' will need to understand her special role as a guide, and be willing to take this task on.

Once a mentor has been chosen, she will need to talk to you as the mother, and together you should decide on the areas of teaching and guidance. Where do you need support, and where does your daughter need more privacy and independence?

The mentor could also play a part in your daughter's special ceremony or celebration.

The following areas are important to growing young women, and need to be addressed at some point in their adolescence. However, they do not all need to be covered by one person alone. A mentor should not feel overwhelmed, but excited, committed and positive about her role.

A 'female curriculum' could include:

General Health

Health foods, exercise, personal hygiene, body image and self-esteem, dieting, bulimia and anorexia, alcohol and drugs.

Menstrual Health

Anatomy and physiology of the female reproductive system, the menstrual cycle, ways to deal with period pains including exercise and the use of natural painkillers like herbs and homeopathy, menstrual hygiene, the use of sanitary protection.

Sexual Health

Female and male anatomy. Girls' and boys' changes during puberty. Information about sex and contraception, healthy relationships, sex and gender identity, sexually transmitted infections, sexual harassment and sexual abuse.

'Herstory'

A look at important women in history and the changing role of women in society. Female role models, including politicians, scientists, artists, musicians and writers, as well as female explorers.

This list is by no means complete and can be added to or changed by mothers, daughters and mentors.

Some areas may be covered at school or addressed at a youth club, whilst many will need to be discussed at home or with a mentor.

Most of all, the mentor acts in the tradition of the 'Wise Woman', who can introduce the girl into the secrets of the female way of life. For you this may include teaching the knowledge of the Goddess, a love for Mother Earth, passing on female rituals, the use of herbs and an awareness of the phases of the moon, and the seasonal cycle of nature.

I hope that you can find a mentor who will help to teach your daughter to learn to love and honour herself and her growing body with wonder and joy.

Teach her to use the bleeding days each month as her creative space, to slow down, to relax, to take extra care of herself, to listen to her dreams, to write, to draw, to walk in nature, to listen to music, to make and create.

Teach her the art of self-love and self-care. Teach her about sisterhood and belonging to the community of women.

May you find your mentor relationship mutually and deeply rewarding!

Contributions (part two)

Red Party - A Mother and Daughter's Story

It all started around St. Valentine's Day, everywhere was red echoing the 'bleeding time', menstruation. Sophie came out the bathroom and told me that she had started to bleed. We hugged and both of us cried. Why? Well, in Sophie's words "I feel happy and sad all together". That best sums up the emotion of the time. It is sad because it signifies the ending of childhood, but, as with any ending, there is also a beginning. Happy because it is the beginning of womanhood.

We therefore wanted to mark this special passage. Sophie had attended some of Anke's workshops, so we decided it was to be a Red Party! We planned it for the next month around the new moon.

For me as the mother of a young woman, it was a time of reflection. I thought about all the women in Sophie's family and mine. About their lives, and the stories I had been told that went to form my view of the world of women.

To reflect this, I made a collage of photographs of all the women in our family, with a picture of Sophie and I at the centre. I am writing their stories, as I know them, to fit into the back of this collage. It is a continuum though; there is room for the next generations of women that will now spring from Sophie.

I also prepared a red box for Sophie, into which I placed

things that had been given to me by these women. A coral necklace from my grandmother, a thimble given to me by a special aunt at my christening, and a pearl ring that my mother gave me. The day of the party approached. Sophie and I had decided that she would spend the night before her celebration with a dear friend, Val. So John and I had the night and day before her celebration alone in preparation for the big event. It really did feel that way; it was very exciting and emotional. We decorated the house with great care, red candles everywhere apart from the sitting room, which was the space for where the ceremony was to begin, so that was decorated with white candles and a single red candle.

When Sophie returned with Val, she looked so different. Val had taken her to the hairdresser who piled her long hair on top of her head. She had returned home a beautiful young woman. I was speechless, so was her father who was also there to greet her. He went shortly afterwards, as it was a female ceremony; he left a poem in her honour. He had also taken her out earlier in the week to buy a special piece of jewellery with a touch of red.

The celebration began as Sophie greeted all the women and girls as they arrived. The girls and women who were menstruating wore some red, those who had not started to bleed wore white, and those who had stopped bleeding wore black. Val lead the ceremony, which is a bit of a blur for me, as I found it hugely emotional. I think it went something like this; we all threaded a bead and spoke a wish for Sophie as she enters womanhood. Some used poems, words from the heart and tears as gifts. Sophie then lit her red candle and from this, lit all the other red candles in the house. We ended the ceremony with a song and presents.

Then on to food! Lots of red food and drinks. The girls disco danced and the women went through as generations before them have 'well in my day!' and 'I remember my first period...' Did we all feel a hundred? Well, maybe in a timeless sense.

John came back from his banishment, sat and chatted; it really was a lovely celebration. One that felt real and creative, not something the card industry has yet to get hold of.

For me the process of reflection goes on and of itself creates new possibilities. On a physical level, my bleeding times were altered by Sophie's, meaning I had two periods one month, another three weeks later. Now we have settled into a rhythm that means we are menstruating together. I also note other changes as I move towards the menopause, the dark of the moon.

Issues of mortality rise, life is not stretching in front of me now as it once did. So, what do I want from this time? Well, I am looking forward to less responsibility for others, more time for myself and growing old disgracefully. You see, to date I have lived a certain story of myself cobbled together, in part, from the stories of the women in my family who came before me. Now I am going to live my own story as it unfolds moment by moment.

So, as Sophie inherits the ability to create life, I create a life of my own.

Fifteen Years later

The ritual was really just the beginning, a doorway through which Sophie passed in the next few years. It was a tough passage as she challenged not only herself but also John and I. Questioning the values and constructs we had put in place to form our family, forcing us to become aware of our vulnerabilities and inconsistencies.

It is a demanding passage, sometimes leaving you on your knees in grief and fear, while at other times brimming with pride and love.

The family narrative shifts and is co-written with our sons and daughters as they take a version of it into the future. Sophie is now 27 years old. She is living and working with her partner Sarah; two beautiful, talented young women who work hard in the digital media business.

John and I are privileged they choose to share so much of their lives with us and I don't know what I would have done without them in the last two years. My mother became terminally ill. Sophie was at my side, and with her support I felt strong enough to carry out mum's last wishes to remain at home until the end. Her dying in this way enabled us to witness her passing: a strange yet beautiful gift. My father died 20 months later, Sophie, and this time Sarah, were at our sides enabling us to fulfil his wish to also die at home.

It was an honour to witness this transition and help prepare the next generation to meet this final task with a diminished sense of fear. Both these rites of passage are part of the cycle of life and should not be hidden, rather celebrated as parts of human experience. When treated in this way they become times of transformation and growth, which makes this book and others like it so important in our ever-changing world.

Fiona Latus

The Sunrise Seed - A Poem from a Father to His Daughter

The strand of life
    flows through
        the very being
            moving towards the whole.
With it, the gift is yours to bring more joy, and
    though the burdens great and
        the responsibilities immense
            the anticipation is hopeful and
                the joy... oh the joy
                    surrounds us all.
In that moment
    you hold life.
It should never
    must never
        will never
            can never
Change.
The seeds for the next phase
    lay firm within the soul.
When the sun rises
The journey begins and
Peace and joy celebrate the future.

                              John Latus

FIRST MENSTRUATION AND BEYOND –
A Mother and Daughter's Story

I have one child, my daughter who is soon to be 17.

She was a happy, bright energetic child and our desire was to educate her along the Steiner small school path. Unfortunately our location in rural Wales only had a Steiner kindergarten which she attended until she followed her friends into the local primary school and then onto the secondary.

Over the years we have struggled to keep open a more creative, intuitive, organic home life against the tide of schoolwork, exams, endless tests and all the accompanying stress.

It was with this background that during her 12th year she began to experience the physical and emotional changes that come with the hormonal upheavals before her first menstruation. It didn't just appear one day, she experienced at various intervals symptoms like headaches, abdominal pains, leg cramps and vaginal discharge.

Delightfully she began bleeding on my birthday! She wanted to stay at home and have a very quiet, gentle day resting, reading and soaking in a lavender bath. In the evening the birthday celebration meal became a first menstruation celebration. It was just our family and her adopted granny who were present.

Over the coming months she needed a lot of support, particularly about the practicalities of menstruation, as at that age it wasn't a topic discussed at all with her friends. Some girls just sail through this time and have no problems adapting to the menstrual rhythm, accommodating it into their lives with ease. It wasn't like this for our daughter.

She has a very slight frame and at 12 was quite faerie-like, almost ephemeral and it was a struggle for her to be in her body and accept these changes as something positive.

Having spent the first part of my own menstrual journey with amenorrhea during A Levels, then experiencing at best mild cramps and at worst horrendous menstruations, I had embarked on a long healing journey to change this pattern. Through naturopathy, meditation, acupuncture, Chinese herbs and personal development work I gained deep insights into the imbalances within me and to the different scenarios these can cause. By the time I became pregnant I had been enjoying my monthly cycle greatly, particularly during the time when I was in the position to blank out my diary to bleed.

I really didn't want my daughter to have the experience I had in those early years and knew I had the knowledge to create the circumstances for her to have a very different journey to mine. I suggested to her that, at the start of her menstruations, she could take two days off school, more if she needed to begin with, to rest, relax, be near a toilet and just have space to experience menstruation as a time to be inward and quiet in the comfort of her own space. To become aware of that inward and downward flow of energy that can be so grounding and re-connecting with the earth's rhythms. That this was not a time to be pushing up and out to achieve in the world of academia and that it was often this energy of pushing that overrides the ease of the menstrual flow and creates tension in the body leading to imbalance and pain.

The following term we did this monthly. My daughter was very regular in a 28 day cycle so it was easy to mark out on the calendar when she would be taking time off. It worked very well and she got much more confident with her bodily changes. It was such a lovely time for us both as we were tending to bleed together.

For six months I would ring up the school and say she was menstruating so would be taking a couple of days off. The school was very good to start with and completely sympathetic when I explained she was getting used to menstruating.

Then my daughter's friends began to ask why she was always taking time off and how bad this was for her work. She was too embarrassed to say it was because of resting while bleeding because she was already marked out as the oddball in school, so she said it was because she was ill.

The school became less tolerant as time went on and GCSE options were chosen, especially with exams looming. Interestingly, the effect this had on me when I made the morning phone call to school, reporting her absence, was to take the easy option and say she was ill with abdominal upsets. I wasn't comfortable with this as I felt it wasn't valuing what we were doing and was giving the impression that there was something wrong with her. However I also accepted that I was a lone voice amongst the teachers, her friends and their parents and this wasn't always easy.

Things came to a head with a very stern letter from the deputy head about my daughter's attendance needing to improve dramatically and a series of telephone calls requesting a home visit from the attendance officer. I was furious about the letter and wrote back laying out exactly what we were doing and why and how much benefit it was having.

She is a highly conscientious A* student. In this sense we were lucky because school could never claim that her work was suffering. She was always helping her friends with their work so they were happy to share with her what she had missed in class. With her it is not "do your homework" but "take a break from your homework".

We did concede that if she began bleeding on days that she had an exam she would attend school and use pain-killers if she needed. But painkillers weren't something she wanted to use on a regular basis to carry on as normal in daily life. In the letter I also mentioned that, practising as a Naturopath for 30 years, I had seen many girls and women in my clinic who never had the opportunity to rest during their menstruation, had pushed through on painkillers and were suffering the consequences of that pattern in later life.

We were fortunate as the letter did strike a chord with the deputy headmistress, and attendance officer, both hav-ing daughters of their own. In fact, individual staff have always been very understanding, it is the education system and its need for statistics that is the issue, this pressure is put on teachers and then passed onto the pupils.

The attendance officer came out to visit us and stayed 2 hours discussing not just my daughter's situation but the need for a change in the general attitude of the education system towards girls and menstruation.

Since this visit we have all come to an agreement that if she needs time off to bleed she takes it and usually she does.

Now five years on from that first menstruation she has a very healthy attitude about bleeding and not pushing at this time, but it has been a lot of work as a mother to get her to this point.

At least now I know she has a choice when she is bleed-ing and the rhythm of resting is well established. On the occasions when it is not possible for her to rest she does resort to some form of pain relief if necessary.

I don't want to give the impression that it was just the time off that helped my daughter. She has also had to make the connection about how her diet and exercise habits affected her menstrual rhythm. Our family diet is good with plenty of fresh vegetables and fruit, not much meat and very low sugar. As a young teen she had her own ideas about chocolate and crisps and would consume a lot, especially the week before bleeding. Her skin would then get very oily and spotty. The result ….a lot of emotional distress. Every month she would question the course of these changes and every month I would give the same reply. Eventually I got frustrated of repeating the same explanation so gave her a challenge. For the following month she would cut down on commercial chocolate and really watch her sugar intake, I would make 'free from' cakes so she still had something sweet to eat. Drink six glasses of water a day and do some exercise daily. She wasn't doing any at school and very little at home, but loves a challenge so agreed to try all this. For the exercise she chose to do a self-help yoga course that she could do in her bedroom after school. The postures and breathing exercises in the course are designed to balance the whole body and are very positive on the hormonal system… and if nothing changed by the end of the month, I would stop the chocolate, water, exercise mantra!

For the next twenty-eight days she took everything on board. She was aware of positive changes a few days into the challenge and this feedback kept her going for the duration. By the end of the month there was a big difference to her skin, the tension in her body, her ability to breathe more fully and she felt more relaxed. It was very empowering for her to understand that the choices she was continuously making in daily life could enable her to create a more balanced lifestyle and that this goes a long way to establishing a healthy menstrual rhythm.

Sarah Hyde

Adolescent Initiation – by a Wise Woman

Adolescence is a wild and exciting and scary time. So many changes, so many unknowns, so much power, such feelings of confusion, mood swings, so much to handle. Sometimes you feel as old as the hills and strong enough to achieve anything. Other times you feel young and irresponsible and just out for a good laugh. Yet again, some people have days when they feel down and hopeless and anxious about how they are going to make it in the world. Who are they anyway, and what sort of a life do they want for themselves? They are supposed to know and they don't.

Adults can seem so out of touch. One's parents can be so outrageously useless. Perhaps this is a time when adults other than one's parents can help with this enormous transition from childhood to womanhood.

This is a time when we encounter dangers and difficulties as we sail through the storm of adolescence after leaving the safe harbour of childhood and before landing on the shores of adulthood. Stories have been told of this time over the years. A good one is 'The Disobedience of the Daughter of the Sun: A Mayan Tale of Ecstasy, Time, and Finding One's True Form', an ancient Guatemalan story that has been written up for us by Martín Prechtel.

In many cultures, special programmes called rites of passage were devised to help girls move from one stage of life to the next. They were created with both the girl and the community in mind so that all could witness the changes she was going through, and they could therefore start treating her differently. Among the Diné, or Navajo, who live in the south-western part of the United States of America, a four day ceremony, the Kinaalda, is held the summer after the girl's first menstruation. During the preparation time the girl is taught her responsibilities as an adult. During the ritual itself, she is transformed into a sacred being: Changing Woman. She is washed, her hair is brushed, she is massaged and dressed in a particular way. She also has her tasks to perform. She has to run every morning and she has to bake a huge cornbread for the whole community. It is hard to give any idea of such an event while just describing the bare bones. But imagine if your whole family, your neighbours, school friends, and teachers were involved. Imagine that you had to work hard but that also you were made to feel special; that you felt a power greater and more extraordinary than yourself, and gradually this overcame you so that for a few days you became shining. The whole world seemed amazing to you, and you seemed amazing to everyone else. In the words of one of the traditional songs sung during the Kinaalda ceremony:

White Shell Girl, they gaze on her...
Now the girl of long life and everlasting beauty,
They gaze on her.
Before her it is beautiful; they gaze on her,
Behind her it is beautiful; they gaze on her...

Everything finishes with a big party, everyone eats some of the cornbread that she has baked, and for a day she is treated as if she were a goddess.

In some cultures, the girls had to face a physical test before they were accepted as adults. On the West Coast of Canada the initiation included a hard swimming race. In another area, there were running races.

In some African countries, and among the First People of Australia also, old customs still survive. In some places initiation was connected to first menstruation. A girl would be hidden away in a special hut or small house once she started to bleed for the first time. Men would be kept away and the women would give her secret teachings. At the end, again she would be brought out and the whole village would throw a big party in her honour.

In Britain we no longer remember what our initiation ceremonies might have been. Some of us are trying to start them up again, borrowing from various traditions around the world.

In 2002 I wrote an article for one of Anke's books about one of my first attempts to help two girls through this transition. I worked with them for a year and they came to visit me every six weeks. They brought me a present and cooked me a meal (which I loved!), and in return I gave them teachings. At the end of the year, they each spent a night out on a Welsh hillside, alone - a brave thing to do. This showed us that they had the courage and the per-severance necessary to take on adult responsibilities. The following morning, when they came down off the hill, they put on dresses that they had made specially, and we feasted and sang for them and every woman present gave them a gift. So they had to work a bit and earn their place. Once they had done that, they were welcomed and fêted and honoured as young women.

Of course, this did not mean they could never be child-like again. Nor that they wanted to leave home. However, they did initiate changes at home to remind themselves and their family that they were no longer children. They took on some new responsibilities and worked out where they were ready to act for themselves.

Since then, I have worked with many young people. For some, just staying out in the woods and keeping awake all night was a great thing. Others have spent a year learning about life and the patterns of the natural world, listening to traditional stories and developing skills like pottery, weaving, knife-making... they then went through a four day initiation and the following year put aside time each week to spend in service to elders.

So an adolescent initiation is a mix of hard work and partying, of earning more freedom by showing that you have developed the courage and stamina necessary for embarking on the life of an adult. And it is a time when you learn how your culture works, how the world around you works, and how you can fit into those patterns in a good way.

Annie Spencer
www.hartwell.eu.com

Further Suggestions for Celebrating Menarche

○ Prepare a moon box or moon basket for your daughter, ready to give to her on her first bleed. You might like to include pads, moontime oil, a moon necklace, a journal, or new underpants. Maybe include a handheld mirror for her to look at her vagina, or you might like to give her an egg stone representing all the eggs in her womb.

○ You could give your daughter a special piece of family jewellery that gets handed on to each younger generation.

○ Or you could buy her a set of Russian dolls, representing her mother-line and give it to her together with photos of each woman.

○ If your daughter does decide to have a celebration, you could use rose petals. Lay out a path of rose petals for her to walk on, use them on your altar, float them in a special bath or use them as a shower of confetti.

○ If you use red candles during the celebration, you could give a small red candle to all the attending girls. Those who have not started yet, could light the candle during their own celebration when the time comes. Those who are bleeding already could light the candle during their next menstruation. The light could be passed on to younger girls.

o You might also like to use red beads during ceremony. Ask each attending girl and woman to bring a red bead that can be strung together into a special necklace. Each bead could be offered with a good wish for your daughter.

o Or you could put together special things that your daughter might like to use each month during her bleed. A moon ring or necklace, a red scarf or red underpants, moontime oil or lovely perfume. Create something that will make your daughter feel special. She will treasure the event and mementos. I am sure she will keep her moon box, basket, or bundle, together with any cards or photos of her celebration.

Afterword

Menarche is a defining moment in our daughter's life. How we welcome her into womanhood will have an enormous impact on her later life. Therefore, we want to make this experience as positive as possible. We want to acknowledge, support, and celebrate her transition.

However, in all this we mustn't forget that this is HER journey! We must try not to impose our ideas and wishes onto her. Our daughters might not want to follow us down the path that we are trying to lead them.

Be prepared for the unexpected. The big day of her first bleed might not turn out as you thought it would. Your daughter might start at a younger age than you expected, and might not be properly prepared for it yet.

She might start on a day when you are too busy and distracted to take in what she is trying to tell you. She might start when she is staying away from home, or she might be too upset about her menarche to feel joyful with you. She might think that she is no longer a child now, and has to be a woman overnight. She might not feel like celebrating.

Whatever situation you will find yourself in, let your daughter know that she is loved and that you are proud of her; that there is no right or wrong way to honour her transition into womanhood.

The best you can do for your daughter is to set a good

example. Learn to live in harmony with your menstrual cycle. Practice self-love and self-care.

In our society we are still a long way away from embracing menstruation. It will take a lot of women to create long lasting change. Hopefully you and your daughter will be part of this movement.

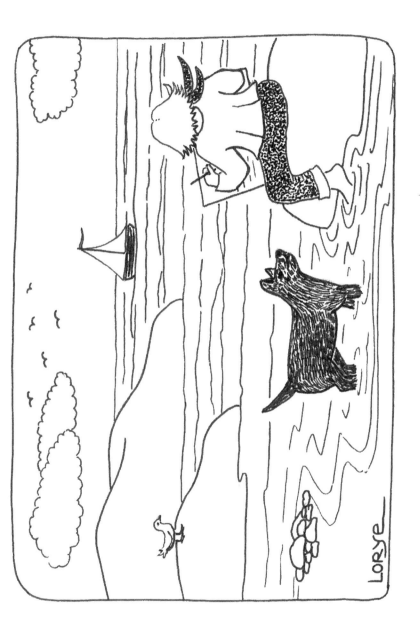

LORYE

Resources

Books for Girls

Reaching for the Moon; a girl's guide to her cycles,
Lucy H. Pearce

The Goddess in You, Patrícia Lemos and Ana Afonso

A Diva's Guide to Getting Your Period, DeAnna L'am

Moon Dreams Diary, Starr Meneely

*Becoming a Woman: A Guide for Girls Approaching
Menstruation,* Jane Hardwicke Collings

*First Moon: Celebration and Support for a Girl's Growing-up
Journey,* Maureen Margaret Smith

Have You Started Yet? Ruth Thomson

What's Happening to Me? Susan Meredith

The Girls' Guide to Growing Up, Anita Naik and Sarah Horne

Soul Searching: A Girl's Guide to Finding Herself,
Sarah Stillman and Susan Gross

The Tapping Solution for Teenage Girls: How to Stop Freaking Out and Keep Being Awesome, Christine Wheeler

Books for Women/Guardians

A Blessing Not a Curse: A Mother-Daughter Guide to the Transition from Child to Woman, Jane Bennett

A Time to Celebrate: A Celebration of a Girl's First Menstrual Period, Jean Morais

A Toolbox for Our Daughters: Building Strength, Confidence and Integrity, Annette Geffert and Diane Brown

Becoming Peers: Mentoring Girls into Womanhood,
DeAnna L'am

Brave Girls: Raising Young Women with Passion and Purpose to Become Powerful Leaders, Stacey Radin

Celebrating Girls: Nurturing and Empowering our Daughters,
Virginia Beane Rutter

Creative Ceremony, Glennie Kindred

Cinderella Ate My Daughter: Dispatches from the Front Lines of the New Girlie-Girl Culture, Peggy Orenstein

Dads and Daughters: How to Inspire, Understand, and Support Your Daughter When She's Growing Up So Fast, Joe Kelly

Daughters of the Moon, Sisters of the Sun: Young Women's Voices on the Transition into Womanhood, K. Wind Hughes and Linda Wolf

From Daughter to Woman: Parenting Girls Safely Through Their Teens, Kim McCabe

Gifts from the Elders: Girls' Path to Womanhood, Gail Burkett

How to Say it to Girls: Communicating with Your Growing Daughter, Nancy Gruver

Menarche: A Journey into Womanhood, Rachael Hertogs

Moon Mother, Moon Daughter: Myths and Rituals that Celebrate a Girls Coming of Age, Janet Lucy and Terry L. Allison

Moon Time: harness the ever-changing energy of your menstrual cycle, Lucy H. Pearce

Mother-Daughter Wisdom: Understanding the Crucial Link Between Mothers, Daughters, and Health, Christiane Northrup

No More Mean Girls: The Secret to Raising Strong, Confident, and Compassionate Girls, Katie Hurley

Puberty Girl, Shushann Movsessian

Raising Girls: How to Help Your Daughter Grow Up Happy, Healthy, and Strong, Steve Biddulph

Red Moon: Understanding and Using the Creative, Sexual and Spiritual Gifts of the Menstrual Cycle, Miranda Gray

Sweet Secrets: Stories of Menstruation,
Kathleen O'Grady and Paula Wansbrough

The Seven Sacred Rites of Menarche: The Spiritual Journey of the Adolescent Girl, Kristi Meisenbach Boylan

The Thundering Years: Rituals and Sacred Wisdom for Teens,
Julie Tallard Johnson

The Wild Genie: The Healing Power of Menstruation,
Alexandra Pope

Wild Girls: The Path of the Young Goddess, Patricia Monaghan

Wild Power: Discover the Magic of Your Menstrual Cycle and Awaken the Feminine Path to Power,
Alexandra Pope and Sjanie Hugo Wurlitzer

Online Resources

www.ritesforgirls.com
Rites for Girls offers mentoring for girls throughout their adolescence. In Girls Journeying Together groups, pre-teen

girls from the age of 10 prepare for puberty and learn how to take charge of their emotional, social, and spiritual well-being. This guidance continues through their teenage years. Rites for Girls also supports mothers, especially while their daughters journey through their teens, and offer training for women who want to learn to facilitate girls' groups.

celebrationdayforgirls.com

This workshop is for girls aged 10-12 years, and their mothers or female carers. It is designed to inspire curiosity, wonder, and appreciation of puberty and the onset of menstruation. The workshop is available in over 20 countries.

www.journeyofyoungwomen.org

Journey of Young Women trains, supports, and connects a global community of mentors who guide girls on their transformative journey to womanhood. Girls are offered circle-based mentoring and rites of passage.

newmoongirls.com

Based in America, they provide support for girls, parents and allies with their New Moon Girls magazine, an online community for girls, and resources for adults.

daughtersoftheearthlodge.com

Daughters of the Earth Lodge are a group of women who work with girls in transition to womanhood. They have a girls' lodge in West Wales, and hold mother and daughter camps for 8-14 year old girls. They also offer a variety of workshops, as well as online mentoring.

talesfromtheeartheart.com

Tales from the Eartheart offer earth wisdom for girls aged 8 years onwards. They offer resources for mentoring girls and holding circles. The website includes ceremonies to download.

wildwise.co.uk

Wildwise offers a programme for girls aged 12-16 years, called 'Wild Time'. It is an annual, nature-based camp on Dartmoor in England. The programme takes place over several weekends and offers girls fun, challenge, and adventure. It allows time and space to explore the connection to self, to each other, and to the earth, and instil a sense of belonging in their bodies, in womanhood, and in nature.

goddessconference.com

The Goddess Conference is an annual international conference held in Glastonbury. Each year it celebrates a different aspect of the many faces of the Goddess. It includes workshops for young people aged 8 - 18 years.

www.moontimes.co.uk

Moon Times sell eco-menstrual products, including organic, washable pads, panty-liners, sponges, and moon cups. They also offer online teachings.

starchild.co.uk

Starchild sells a 'Moon Time' massage oil. It contains a soothing blend of essential oils to help relax and release stress and discomfort during menstruation.

redschool.net

The Red School offers online courses based on a radical new approach to menstruation, from menarche to menopause. It teaches about the power of the menstrual cycle and awakening menstruality consciousness.

redtenttemplemovement.com

This is a grass-roots movement for women of all ages that has spread worldwide over the last decade. A red tent is a place to take time out during our bleeding days, a place to go inward and share with other women. It is a place where you can honour your body and your cycle. Moon lodges originate from the Native American tradition. They honoured the moontime as sacred and it was treated with respect. Menstruation was seen as a time for dreaming and visioning.

dianafabianova.com/moon-inside-you-movie

A film on menstruation by Diana Fabianova, 'The Moon Inside You,' explores menstrual etiquette with doses of humour and self-irony, the documentary approaches the subject through both personal and collective references, thus challenging our preconceived idea of womanhood.

Acknowledgements

With special thanks to Jaine Raine, Miranda Hartwell, Lorye Keats Hopper, Wendy Andrew, Lucy H. Pearce, and Patrick Treacy. All the women who have supported First Moon since 2000, and all those who have contributed to this new edition. Cora Paine, Sarah Hyde, Fiona and John Latus, Annie Spencer, Sandra Bruce, Gabrielle O'Connell, and Avena Rawnsley.

About the Cover Artist

Wendy Andrew lives, dreams and paints in the beautiful countryside on the Wiltshire/Dorset border.

Her paintings are inspired by the ancient mysteries that are wrapped in the turning of the seasons and the natural rhythms of life that give pattern to our being.

www.paintingdreams.co.uk

About the Illustrator

Lorye Keats Hopper works with the creative healing arts. She has facilitated and guided women's healing retreats for many years and also worked with young people in schools, youth clubs, and international youth conferences.

About the Author

Anke Mai has always been passionate about girls' empowerment. She has been a feminist since her early teens and was active in the women's movement in Germany throughout her teenage years. She believes in giving girls the freedom and encouragement to be themselves. Anke is the mother of two grown-up daughters and has worked with girls in many different settings over the years.

www.ankemai.co.uk

The front cover artwork is available as a card from Anke, together with other beautiful cards for girls.

References

i.   *Celebrating Girls,* Virginia Beane Rutter, Conari Press.

ii.   *Red Moon Passage,* Bonnie J. Horrigan, Thorsons.

iii. *The Woman's Encyclopaedia of Myths and Secrets,*
Barbara Walker, Harper and Row.

Women's Medicine Ways, Marcia Starck,
The Crossing Press.

Der Mondring, Margaret Minker, dtv Verlag.

Printed in Poland
by Amazon Fulfillment
Poland Sp. z o.o., Wrocław